# LIFE LESSONS FOR HEALTHCARE WORKERS

*The Ones You Might Not Learn in School*

DR. MICHAEL GUMUKA

I0210049

# LIFE LESSONS FOR HEALTHCARE WORKERS

*Special Thanks to Christina and Sean.*

Copyright © 2021 by Michael Gumuka.

All rights reserved. No part of this book may be reproduced in any manner whatsoever without written permission except in the case of brief quotations embodied in critical articles and reviews.

While every precaution has been taken in the preparation of this book, the publisher assumes no responsibility for errors or omissions, or for damages resulting from the use of the information contained herein.

ISBN: 978-1-7368329-1-2

Written by Michael Gumuka.

First Printing, 2021.

# Contents

FINAL THOUGHTS

CREDITS

# Introduction

My name is Mike. On the job, I go by 'Dr. Mike'. I have been a physician for years, and I have seen some significant changes in healthcare since I graduated from school. I have worked in primary care, with all of its trials and tribulations, and in urgent care, which has its own problems. These fields are opposites in many ways, but medicine is still medicine. In this book, I will try to provide insight into some life lessons that I have learned on my journey to help future generations of health care workers (of all levels, not just physicians) provide better care and have better lives. I hope to reach providers, nurses, technicians, receptionists, janitors, couriers, and students – everyone on the healthcare team. Remember – healthcare is a team sport, and the team is only as strong as its members and the teamwork/communication between them.

After going through high school, college, medical school, and residency, I have gotten pretty tired of homework. Since I would love to think that this book will find a home in classrooms someday, I have tried to keep it as short, sweet, and to the point as possible (you're welcome!).

Over the years, I have done a lot of teaching in medicine. I take students of all levels regularly, visit high school classrooms every year, and provide a fair amount of on-the-job training. The lessons and stories I present here have all been selected to show specific points – and make those points memorable. While most of these examples are inspired by true stories, *all* of them have been adapted for educational purposes. Any details (age, gender, etc.) added are fictional, and their sole purpose is to make the stories easier to read. I do not believe that altering these stories will impact the value of the life lessons I present, but it will certainly protect everyone's privacy. To reiterate, no *actual* patients or cases will be presented here. Any similarities to actual people (living or deceased) is purely coincidental. No identification with actual people (living or deceased) is intended or should be inferred.

So, without further ado...here are my best lessons. Good luck to everyone reading this book, wherever you may be, and however you care for people.

PS – To give credit where it's due, many of these lessons were taught to me by various attendings, residents, and students over the years. I have simply tried to condense them all into one source.

PPS – I would like to formally state that these are only my opinions and experiences, not consensus or facts. It is not my intent to offend anyone or imply that my way of thinking is the only way. Please enjoy this book for what it is, and like most things in life, take it with a grain of salt.

# I

## Students Matter!

This point is so overlooked that it's nauseating. In healthcare, the student is always the one who feels like the dumbest person in the room (even though they're not). The way rotations are scheduled (usually 4-6 weeks at each location), there's usually just enough time to start feeling like you understand your duties before having to start a new rotation, often in an entirely different specialty. For med students, at least, this process lasts for two years. Then in residency, it is repeated for at least another three years. That is a *five-year period* of constantly being the new person, who doesn't have a good handle on their job, and is continuously trying to adapt to new roles and responsibilities. It is staggering how burned out you can get when you feel like you are always the dumbest one in the room.

As a quick aside, when you are going through your clinical rotations or starting a new job, you are not the *dumbest* person in the room, just the *newest*. I learned this at the start of my second year of residency. The new interns (a special term for first-year residents – I am convinced that doctors make up extra words to sound smarter) had just arrived, and they were hopelessly lost. They didn't know where the bathrooms were, where the kitchen was, how to find the right hospital forms for admissions or discharges, or even how to page the specialists during rounds. None of these things required medical training, just experience. After a single year, I had all of these processes down to a science. Then we started talking about medicine, and it became even *more* apparent that I had learned a lot. Watching the new graduates made me feel better about myself. I'm not bragging; it was reassuring to know I wasn't hopeless and see how far I had come in a single year. I made a point of teaching them everything I could, and I stopped letting myself feel dumb.

Now, back to students being important. In the workforce, speed matters. You will be pushed to do your job as fast as you can without making mistakes. The farther along you are in your training, the truer this becomes – but no one is worried about your speed as a student. That makes students a precious resource because they can sit with a complicated patient and connect with them as people, making it much easier for patients to 'open up' about their problems. I can remember at least half a dozen cases where hospitalized patients (who had been seen by multiple doctors, nurses, and therapists) weren't properly diagnosed until a student found the missing details in a history.

Patients often have pretty strong feelings about students, seeing them as an inconvenience, something to be 'put up with' at a teaching hospital. In reality, students are some of the kindest and most gentle people on the team. They still have a 'save the world complex,' and they don't rush due to time constraints. Smart patients will specifically ask for students. A patient once told me that he wouldn't consent to a procedure unless I had a student perform it, because he felt students were gentler. I didn't get offended; I had a student assist me. It was a great teaching opportunity, and an excellent reminder of how much students matter to patients.

People often learn best by 'doing.' Obviously, this includes healthcare students. There are many ways to teach students, but my personal favorite involves giving them some real responsibility. For example, asking a student, "What would you treat Susan's strep throat with?" is a purely academic exercise. Whether they get it right or wrong, the teacher will still take care of 'Susan.' I once had a student for several months, and I grew confident in her abilities, so one day I told her to see 'Susan' and decide on an antibiotic. I also told her that no matter what she chose, I would send in the script before I saw Susan myself.

Interestingly, my student took twice as long as she usually did to see Susan. She struggled for almost 20 minutes before settling on a script for antibiotics (I made her pick the dose and duration for treatment, too). I then sent the script to the pharmacy *before* seeing the patient. What I didn't tell my student at the time was that I had already gone through the chart, checked Susan's allergies and med list, and spoken with Susan briefly, and knew the script was a good choice – Susan was never in any danger of being given a 'wrong' script. It was a great learning experience. After the visit, when my student asked me if her choice was the right one, I said, "We'll find out soon enough...hopefully, she doesn't die." My poor student called Susan later that week to make sure everything was going well (and it was).

I continued to have my student pick the scripts like this for certain cases (ones I knew she could handle), and soon she was so comfortable looking up any information she needed that she no longer needed my help. Months later, when she was applying for residency, one of the program directors asked me if she was ready. I told him, quite honestly, that I would have felt comfortable handing her my pager. She knew what to do, and if she didn't know, she would either look up the information she needed or call me directly. (Note – I never actually gave her my pager. Pointing that out for legal purposes.)

Teaching will also keep your skills sharp. I have had to review or learn new skills over the years to help students with special interests. Answering their questions will make you review information you haven't seen in years and keep you up to date with new practices. Sometimes students are learning things in school that you aren't familiar with, and they can teach *you* a few things. Most of the time, you don't tell them that, of course, but it's just another example of how valuable students can be to you, as well as your patients.

# 2

## The Point of Ethics Class

Ethics class. Everyone's favorite – long discussions, weird hypothetical scenarios, and subjective test questions. What's not to love? On paper, ethics class teaches people how to be 'morally upright' in their field. In reality, ethics class probably isn't going to change anyone. Let's face it – if you're a jerk before ethics class, you'll probably still be a jerk after it. So what's the point, then? And why does everyone have to go through it?

I believe ethics class makes people *think*. At least once during the course, there will be some issue or dilemma that bothers you. Maybe it's a medical issue or a legal loophole. Perhaps it's a social issue you've never encountered. The emotions generated by your discussions in class will drive you to form an opinion. As the course goes on, being exposed to multiple perspectives will help you refine your opinion - and now you've *thought* about something. Mission accomplished.

The key to ethics class is to learn how to 'zoom out' during challenging situations, which occur almost every week in healthcare. Let me give you an example. I once cared for a man who was critically ill. He was in the hospital for almost a week before he died. When he first arrived at the hospital, he was diagnosed with septic shock (a severe blood infection). His male partner of many years was at his bedside. They were not legally married (this was before same-sex marriage was legalized), but they were *practically* married, and his partner had been caring for him for a long, long time. As the emergency room staff were checking him in, they completed a MOLST form – a set of legal orders that guide end-of-life care. These orders also allow you to designate a health care proxy – someone you want to make decisions for you, in case you can't make them for yourself (like when you're unconscious). The patient had signed the form, and so had his partner. There were two witness signatures required, but in the confusion of getting this man admitted and transferred to the intensive care unit (ICU), only *one* witness signed it. It didn't matter for the first few days – we all knew the patient's wishes, and we spoke to his partner about medical decisions.

The problem arose when his family found out he was in the hospital. The patient hadn't spoken to his family in years because they disapproved of his male life-partner. Even though they had virtually disowned our patient, they came to his bedside when they learned he was hospitalized, claiming the right to make his medical decisions as his next of kin. They also threatened to sue anyone who spoke to the partner.

Situations like these are an unfortunate example of the tragedy that can occur when ethics and the law are at odds.

We have a piece of paper, signed by our unconscious and dying patient, declaring his partner as his healthcare proxy. His family (who ostracized our patient and hated his partner) is ready to sue us if we provide any information to his partner. According to the hospital's legal team, the entire MOLST form was considered invalid because a witness signature was missing. Ultimately, the family was allowed to direct our patient's care, and the partner was not given any medical updates, though he was still allowed to visit per hospital policy. This unfortunate, loving man had to learn about his partner's death in the obituaries.

Here's another example with the same type of scenario. A young woman was admitted to the hospital, transferred to the ICU, and was eventually declared brain-dead. Her family had been contacted, and they were coming into town. Her boyfriend, whom she had been living with for decades, was extremely devoted. He rarely left her bedside. When her family arrived, they had the legal right to make decisions for her as next of kin, since no healthcare proxy had been named, and she wasn't married. Her family made it clear that her boyfriend could visit per hospital policy but could not receive updates on her status. Apparently, her family never approved of our patient's interracial relationship.

When the woman was declared brain-dead, her family wanted her to be an organ donor, and it took a few days to perform all of the necessary tests. These included scans for cancer, blood tests for things like HIV or hepatitis, etc. According to her boyfriend, our patient had voiced a preference *not* to be an organ donor. Unfortunately, there were no *written* advanced directives in place, so we had no choice but to proceed according to the family's wishes. To make things worse, because the family had forbidden us from updating her boyfriend, he had no idea she was technically dead. The same day she was taken off life support and transferred for organ harvesting, he was at her bedside, talking to her and holding her hand, looking forward to being with her again. I was on call that night, making my rounds. When he asked me if she was going to wake up, I told him that I wasn't allowed to update him. I had no choice. I apologized, and I meant it. When he left that night, I cried. Right in the hospital. We'll talk about that later. For now, the big question is, what does this have to do with ethics class?

Remember, the point of ethics class is to make you think about *all* sides of a situation. In the examples above, I make it pretty clear how I feel – the families were the bad guys in both cases. Trying to ostracize someone based on gender, orientation, or race is wrong – especially when their only crime is being loving and supportive. However, not every case is about race or sex. Sometimes it's just a personality clash. In those cases, there may not be an easily identifiable 'bad guy.' For example, when an older adult is at the end of life, ready to move forward with comfort care, it is relatively common to have mixed reactions from their family members. Relatives from out of town aren't ready to say goodbye. The ones that live locally are exhausted and at peace with comfort care because they have done everything they can to help. As the patient moves forward with comfort care, though, the family members from out of town often feel guilty about 'not being there' and want more time. Accusations sometimes start to fly because everyone is exhausted, grieving, and upset. Families can be torn apart by these arguments. Unfortunately, I have seen it happen.

I once cared for a dying woman with several daughters, one of whom lived several hours away. While most of the children were comfortable with mom being on comfort care, the daughter from out of town (we'll call her Susie) was quite loud in her objections. During the time I was caring for their mother, I had witnessed multiple arguments between the siblings. Susie would repeatedly accuse her sisters of killing her mother. I finally asked Susie (in private) if she was truly angry at her sisters, explaining that relatives from out of town often feel guilty about 'not being around' or feel angry at their parents for dying. I also reassured her that these were normal parts of the grieving process. I told her there was no reason to feel guilty about her mother's comfort care, and she should use the time she had left to make peace with her family members instead of being angry at them. When she finished cursing and swearing at me (and threatening me with lawsuits), she stormed out of the room. The next day, though, she came and apologized. The family ended up doing really well after that. In hindsight, there are gentler, more compassionate ways to say the things I said that day. My skills have improved since then. As for ethics class? It helped me 'zoom out' and realize the angry sister in this example wasn't the bad guy. She was suffering and grieving in her own way, and as long as I kept that in mind, I was able to help her. Pay attention in ethics class – it will help in ways you never expect.

On a final note, not all ethical dilemmas involve end-of-life care. This chapter could easily have included examples about abortions, addiction, domestic abuse, or privacy issues.

Here's a quick example: I once cared for a young girl who had been hospitalized for social issues. She had been trading sex for drugs – with her *cousin*. Since she was a minor, she couldn't consent to her own treatment. My team and I weren't sure who had the authority to make decisions for her because CPS (Child Protective Services) had removed the child from her parents. Even if we *had* a clear decision-maker, none of us were comfortable discharging her until she had a stable home. While the medical aspects of this case were pretty straightforward, the social, ethical, and legal issues were mindboggling. Thank goodness for ethics class, right?

# 3

## Preparing for Life After School

Everyone has their own definition of 'adulthood.' These range from being 18 years old to graduating from school to being financially independent. Whatever your definition, at some point you are going to have to be financially responsible for yourself, and possibly others, too. Just having a job isn't enough – you also have to manage your money well. There are many books and guides available on how to do that, so I will just provide some basic advice for healthcare workers.

Many healthcare workers go to college before having their first 'real' job. They live on a tight budget for years, sometimes using loans as their only source of income. When the day finally comes that they get a decent paycheck, sometimes they go a little crazy. I strongly recommend living your first year with a real job in the same lifestyle you had as a student.

In other words, don't buy a new car, or a new house, or a whole new wardrobe. Use the same clunky vehicle you have had for years. Find a reasonably cheap apartment. Use hand-me-down or used furniture. Even though you now have more money than ever before, you probably have some serious student loans. Many of my colleagues were still paying off their student loans when their children were getting ready for college! Imagine trying to pay for a mortgage, a car, and college expenses for yourself *and* your child at the same time! That doesn't even count 'luxuries' like food, gas, electricity, or clothes.

My first few years after residency were spent in a somewhat smelly apartment building, with no new furniture and a nearly ten-year-old car. However, I paid off a large portion of my loans (almost half of them) in that time. Later on, as I got married, had kids, and bought a house (and a dog!), I was able to keep chipping away at my loans, paying them off 10-11 years after graduating from residency. It was amazing how hard it was to make real progress on them once I had a family. If you have the chance to pay your loans down before making any major purchases, do it. You won't regret it.

Now that we have mentioned marriage and families, here's a little-known fact: There's a chance that if you get married before you get a professional license, your spouse will own half of your license. You'll need to check the latest laws to be sure. The legal reasoning (I think) is that your spouse likely had to make sacrifices in order for you to get your license, so they deserve some of the income from that license (in case of divorce, etc.). If you aren't married yet, whether you're licensed or not, think about a prenup. Prenups (prenuptial agreements) protect both you and your spouse in case of divorce. Considering the divorce rate in our country, this should be a no-brainer. It doesn't mean you aren't serious about marriage and commitment – it just means you're smart. Think about it like this: You always get your car inspected and buckle your seatbelt, but you also get car insurance and life insurance, right? Even though you hope it never matters. Same idea here – it's just smarter to get the prenup.

Buying a house or a car doesn't need to be a fashion statement. You don't need status symbols just because you have a medical degree. It's okay to have nice things, but after years and years of working to get to a point where you have some money to work with, don't spend it all trying to have the best of everything. Having 'average' quality belongings and very little stress is *way* better than having top-notch stuff and desperately trying to pay for it all. Money is just a tool, after all, to buy food, shelter, and clothes. It won't make you happy by itself. Use it to help make great memories: Go on vacation. Spend time with your family. Make some friends. Find a hobby. Here's an idea –sit down and relax for a while. Smell the flowers. Seriously – try *literally* smelling the flowers the next time you go walking outside. It's amazing.

# 4

## The Three Rules of Medicine

Rule 1: Eat when you can.

Rule 2: Sleep when you can.

Rule 3: Go when you can (yes, I mean the restroom).

Rule 4: Don't mess with the pancreas (surgeons only).

Surgeons like to feel special, and they get a lot of grief for it in the medical world, but here it is in writing: They deserve it. Their training is *hard*. Their lifestyle is *hard*. Being on call as a surgeon is *hard*. So yes, they are allowed to have an extra rule. They also deserve some extra respect, even though they aren't *actually* perfect (just don't point that out to them directly...it might not end well).

One would think that with all of our knowledge as healthcare workers, our three main rules would involve being diligent, protecting privacy, and being compassionate. However, our three most important rules are actually about taking care of ourselves. While this might seem ironic, it's disturbing just how often we neglect ourselves on the job.

Medical shifts tend to start early and end late. Whether inpatient (hospitals, nursing homes, places that need staffing 24 hours per day) or outpatient (the usual doctor's offices, etc.), a 40-hour workweek is a luxury. If you're in residency, your weeks will likely be 80 hours long, at least. Residents get pushed so hard that laws have been passed to prevent extreme exhaustion. Lawmakers finally realized that when doctors work 120 hours per week, patients tend to die more often. However, 80 hours per week is still rough, and trying to cram 120 hours' worth of work into an 80-hour week means everyone has to move even faster than usual. That's why medical workers tend to forget to eat, drink, or use the restroom. They are trying so hard to help everyone else (as fast as they can) that they forget to take care of themselves.

If you think about it, a half-starved, dehydrated, constipated health care worker with a UTI (urinary tract infection) and sleep deprivation is *not* the kind of caregiver you want when you're sick. Besides, the odds of someone dying, being mistreated, or even just getting mad if you take a 20-minute break for lunch are pretty low. As hard as it is to accept, no single one of us is so important that the medical system would crash if we ate lunch. Even surgeons can take the time to eat – and the operating room literally *can't* run without them. So please, remember to eat lunch and dinner, even if you are working. Stay hydrated. If you have to use the restroom, do it. There won't be a 'good' time, which means there won't be a 'bad' time. Just go. It's going to be okay.

Let's talk about Rule #2: Sleep when you can. This rule is primarily for providers since nurses, techs, and receptionists don't usually work 24-hour shifts. Sleeping on the job can be crucial when you're on call, so find a good place (a call room, your home, the hospital library, wherever) where you can sleep for an hour or two if you get the chance. Even if you feel good on a particular shift, these long hours will take their toll on you over time. There's nothing wrong with telling the nurses you need to sleep. They will often work with you, as long as you are polite about it. When you can't take the time to sleep, eat something. Calories make a good substitute for sleep, but only once in a while. At one point, I could devour a small pizza and a soda and be wide awake for about 4-5 hours. That kind of eating will make you *really* unhealthy if you do it too often, so use it as a last resort, and sleep when you can.

# 5

## The Power of Words

Finally, we can start talking about the good stuff! A wise man once told me that no one goes to the doctor's office unless they're scared. Period. Even the gruff old man who insists he only came in today because 'his wife made him' is afraid of something (even if it's his wife). Try to keep that in mind when you talk to people. To give credit where it's due, the man who taught me this was one of my medical school professors, who taught us about the *art* of medicine, in addition to the science.

Words can be used to both help and hurt people, sometimes unintentionally. We've all said the wrong thing at the wrong time. However, as healthcare workers dealing with scared patients, our words take on enormous power. As cliché as it sounds, that gives us a great responsibility. No one's perfect, but we need to think about our words more carefully than most. Let me give you some examples.

Early in my career, one of my hospitalized patients was dehydrated and had a urinary infection. While these two things often occur together, this patient was a young man. Urinary infections are much less common in males, so I worked him up more thoroughly. Part of the workup involved an ultrasound of his kidneys. The test was essentially normal; he had some slight variations that were within normal limits, but no real pathology. I tried to explain this to his anxious mother, but she was *not* happy that his ultrasound was 'essentially' normal. She wanted to know why it wasn't 'totally' normal – and what I planned to do about it. The more I tried to explain that her son's kidneys were fine, the angrier she became. She thought I was trying to cover something up. I tried to explain how ultrasound works (using soundwaves to generate a picture), then I tried to explain what 'incidental findings' were. I tried everything. She just kept getting more anxious and angry.

After about five minutes of letting me dig myself into a hole, my attending physician put his hands on my shoulders and said, "What my young friend here is trying to say is that everyone's kidneys are different, kind of like fingerprints. What radiology saw was just normal variation and is absolutely nothing to be worried about." The effect was immediate – mom settled right down and asked why I hadn't just said that in the first place. My attending's response was perfect: "Because he's been a doctor for three days and is still learning the important things." We all had a good laugh at my expense, and I made the words 'normal variation' a permanent part of my vocabulary. You should, too.

My favorite example of the power of words involves a new

mom in a parking garage. It was winter, and there was snow on the ground. I had just finished a 24-hour shift on labor and delivery and was finally heading home for some sleep. There was a bridge that connected the hospital to the parking garage, and as I was leaving, I saw someone crying to herself at the edge of the parking area. She was still hooked up to an IV pole, with fluids running. As it turned out, it was one of my patients from that night. She was crying outside in the snow, dressed in little more than a hospital gown, with an IV running, within hours of delivering a child. She didn't know I was there, and it would have been easy to keep walking (at this point, there was nothing between me and my pillow at home). After a few seconds of wrestling with myself, I went over and asked her what was wrong. Obviously, in hindsight, I know that talking to her was the right thing to do, but after being awake for nearly 30 hours straight, I wasn't exactly thinking clearly.

It turned out she was crying because she felt like the worst mom in the world. She had called CPS and asked them to check on her other kids at home. She had had issues with post-partum depression in the past, and was afraid she wouldn't be able to care for her kids appropriately. As she put it, what kind of mom has to call CPS on herself? She had become a new mom again just a few hours ago and was already at the lowest point she could imagine. She couldn't handle any more shouts of 'Congratulations!' from nurses, friends, family, and everyone else in the hospital – it all felt fake to her, which is why I found her crying outside in the snow.

When she finished telling me her story, I was silent for a moment, weighing my next words carefully. I had already learned the power of words. I told her that I understood what she was saying, but I saw things very differently than she did. I felt she was one of the best moms I'd ever met. Calling CPS on herself was incredibly brave and a huge risk. I explained that CPS *exists* because so many children are abused, neglected, or both. The problem is so common that our government had to set up a special unit just to help all of these kids. Most parents are terrified of CPS, so to be able to put her own feelings and pride aside and ask for help for her children, knowing there was a risk of losing her children...that's love. Truly selfless love. The kind only a great parent could show. (Okay, yes – by this point, I was trying not to cry, too.) Seeing the look on her face as she thought about what I said, to realize she had nothing to be ashamed of, was an experience that will stay with me forever. It only took 10-15 minutes of my time, and this young woman was able to smile, be proud of herself, and walk back into the hospital to see her baby. I never saw her again, but I am confident she continues to be a great mom to this day.

# 6

## The Poker Face

Everyone has been in awkward situations, no matter what their career. In healthcare, though, these situations come up pretty often. The important thing to remember? Don't judge. It's harder than you think. A drug addict comes in after their third overdose this week? Help them. Someone has nightmares and anxiety after they crashed a car while driving drunk? Help them. A longtime patient shows up for a routine physical exam the day after their spouse informs you they are being abused? Help them. You can't judge or condemn. All you can do is help the person in front of you.

On a lighter note, the poker face is equally important when you hear something comical, like the time someone from animal control came in because they 'lost a wrestling match with a raccoon.' How about a newly-wed couple that came in because the husband 'cut his wrist' and was 'bleeding out.' His wife was sobbing, but when we finally unwrapped the wound, it was a scratch. Seriously - we just put a band aid on it. In times like these, laughing at someone just makes them feel small, which is not acceptable. However, in the interest of good storytelling, I have some examples for you. Some of these are hilarious, some are disturbing, but all of these situations required a poker face.

I once took care of a young woman who had been vomiting for weeks, mainly in the morning. She told the nurses ahead of time that she was pregnant. She was worried about morning sickness, but her mother didn't know she was pregnant, and the patient (we'll call her Jane) wanted to keep it that way. In the exam room, Jane was on the exam table, and Mom was in a chair behind her. Mom immediately asked how far along Jane was in her pregnancy (mom had suspicions, apparently). At that moment, Jane leaned in and started rapidly blinking her left eye at me. Only her left eye. I soon realized this was her way of telling me something was 'up.' Mom then explained that Jane went into labor last month, was starting to dilate, but hadn't had her baby yet. Quick medical lesson: when a woman is in labor and begins to dilate, birth will happen within 1-2 days in almost every case. It will *never* last a month. Ever. When I explained this to Mom, Jane started blinking at me as fast as she could again (still only with the left eye). Imagine trying to keep a straight face, keep a secret, dodge questions, and provide Mom with education while being blinked at like that!

Eventually, we got mom out of the room, had an open conversation, and treated Jane's morning sickness. We set her up for prenatal care, too. Her mom didn't find out she was pregnant that day. I tried to get Jane to realize that she would have to tell her mom about the pregnancy sooner or later. I even offered to help deliver the news, but she wasn't interested. The funniest part of this whole story? Jane was an adult! Mom didn't even need to be there.

Some people have the most annoying habit of coming in to be seen within minutes of closing time. If we close at 5 pm, they show up at 4:50 pm. Closing at 8 pm? They show up at 7:55 pm. When people show up at the last minute because of an acute injury, something that just happened, I don't get upset. When it's because of something that started days or weeks ago, it bothers me, but I can't show it. One night, just before we closed, a woman came running (yes, *running*) into the office because she couldn't breathe. She was a former smoker who had switched to vaping. That night, though, she had read an article that said vaping was still unhealthy. She panicked, decided she couldn't breathe anymore, and came in for evaluation. In this case, her anxiety was reasonable, if over-dramatic. During our conversation, she was entirely rational. The part that was hard to handle was her shirt. It said, "Suck it up, Buttercup."

One last example before we move on: A man came in for a 'personal problem.' He was angry, cursing, and swearing because he had developed genital warts, which are transmitted sexually. He was upset with the (multiple) women he was sleeping with for giving him warts. We talked about safe sex practices, which he wasn't interested in, and decided to do some blood work to look for other sexually transmitted infections. Since the lab was closing soon, I asked the technicians to draw his blood in the exam room. Two of them went in together (both female), and while they were drawing his blood, he tried to flirt with them. Remember – we're not allowed to judge. Even the two lab techs had to be polite while they ignored his advances.

Good luck with your poker face, everyone. You'll need it.

# 7

## Trust Your Gut

Medicine is not a perfect science. We estimate that about half of what we know is wrong at any given time – we just don't know which half. As research continues and technology improves, we are continually making new discoveries, revisiting old theories, and developing new treatments. With all the uncertainty in medical science, it can be hard to know what to believe and which sources to trust. That's where your gut comes in. Always trust your gut.

I was taught, and I teach all my students, that the single most crucial part of the physical exam is your overall gestalt – the immediate impression you get when you look at someone. Are they okay or not? If someone looks bad (sick, short of breath, shaky and pale, etc.), and you can't find anything wrong with them, then you need to keep looking, even if it means sending them to a higher level of care. You won't be right every time. I'm not. I have sent plenty of people to the emergency room, only to find out there was nothing seriously wrong, and that's okay. I would much rather have people evaluated than risk someone's life by not trusting my gut. For the record, I've also *saved* quite a few lives by sending people to the emergency room.

I once sent a child to a hospital, about 20 minutes away, during a blizzard. Her history and exam were classic for appendicitis, which is an emergency. Even though the roads were slick, her parents drove her to the emergency room. Soon after that, one of the ER doctors called to yell at me because I sent someone to the hospital during a blizzard for 'rib pain.' After letting him yell at me for 2-3 minutes, I asked him if he had examined the patient yet. When he didn't answer, I told him that if he *examined* her abdomen, he would find right lower quadrant tenderness, with guarding and rebound tenderness, as well as a positive psoas sign – all of which point to appendicitis. I then told him that when he found those things, he should call the surgeon, and he should do his job before calling to yell at me next time. I never heard back from the ER doctor, but the girl had surgery that afternoon. By trusting my gut, even in the face of adversity, I saved her life that day.

Years ago, a woman brought her son (we'll call him Bob) to the office to refill his asthma medications. I had seen them both before but never knew Bob had asthma. When I examined him, his lungs sounded perfect. There was no evidence of asthma on exam – or in his medical records. When I pointed this out to his mother, she became outraged. I tried to explain that not having asthma was a *good* thing, and even if children sometimes need an inhaler when they are sick, it doesn't mean they have asthma (though it may increase the risk of developing it later). Mom wasn't having it and started demanding a nebulizer machine. I was reluctant to order one because it wasn't necessary. She threatened to sue me if I didn't give Bob a nebulizer, so I told her I would check with their previous pediatrician, and if Bob needed an inhaler, I would order it.

Interestingly, Bob's prior healthcare provider was not aware of any asthmatic issues. As a result, I did not order a nebulizer. Mom never sued me, but I soon received a letter from the electric company stating that Mom hadn't paid her bill in months. They wanted me to confirm that Bob needed a nebulizer. Since Mom had claimed her son had asthma and needed a nebulizer to survive, the power company couldn't legally deny her electricity. When I would not confirm the need for a nebulizer, Mom had to pay her power bill. In this case, Mom's original request was pretty reasonable – healthcare providers refill medications every day. However, her response to my questions was very unusual, leading to my suspicions about her motives.

As a quick aside – labeling children as asthmatic for free electricity (besides being illegal) puts them on a lifelong path of being 'sick.' Schools will presume they need inhalers, or special treatment in gym class, when no accommodations are necessary or appropriate.

Okay, one last example for this chapter. Sometimes it takes a few visits to get to the bottom of a complicated case. Fair warning – this story gets pretty ridiculous.

I had the opportunity to see a young lady several times within a year. We'll call her Jane, to make things easier. Jane had been having constant belly pain for months. No one could figure out why. She had been to multiple specialists, and her workup was always completely normal. The first time I examined Jane, I started her on antacids and advised her to increase her intake of fluids and fiber. I was upfront about the fact that I had very little to add to her workup. After a while, Jane came back to see me again. Her symptoms were getting worse. Her workup had been repeated and was still normal. I asked her if she had any new life stressors – relationship issues, school problems, etc. Stress is a *very* common cause of gut-related symptoms. Jane and her mother were both adamant that there were no new stressors at home (which was a clear indicator to me that there was a big one), but neither of them would say anything, and they left the office.

A few months later, I saw Jane a third time. She was still complaining of abdominal pain. This time, I didn't even bother with a physical workup. I was pretty convinced, based on a gut feeling, that her symptoms were stress-related. After over 30 minutes of questioning, Jane and mom finally opened up. Jane's symptoms had begun soon after she found out her boyfriend was cheating on her – with her *mom*. When Jane confronted her mother, Mom decided that 'open communication' would be best. Mom had been sharing the text messages between herself and the boyfriend with Jane, including 'sexting' messages (sexually explicit messages and photos). Understandably, seeing romantic messages and photos involving her mother and her boyfriend caused a lot of stress for Jane, which was the source of her abdominal pain. Ultimately, I am not aware of how their social situation worked out, but I sent them to see psychiatry. The whole family needed some serious counseling.

# 8

## Staying Open-Minded

I have found the most stereotypical thing about people is that they hate being stereotyped. In medicine, though, we tend to stereotype a lot. Sometimes this can be helpful – after all, common things occur commonly. Knowing the common presentations of illnesses or injuries can save a lot of time on busy days. However, just as stereotypes are not always accurate, the common solutions to medical complaints are not always right, either. For example, the teenager who is repeatedly falling asleep in school and states they just aren't sleeping well could be lazy. Or they could be experimenting with drugs. Are they sneaking out at night? Do they have undiagnosed heart disease? Or sleep apnea? I've seen most of these issues in my career – and they have all had similar presentations.

I once had a teenager come in with his mother complaining that he was tired all the time. The issue had been present for several weeks. Since he was a teenager, I interviewed him twice (with and without his mother present). When she left, the patient (John, to make storytelling easier) told me he was involved with a new girlfriend, who liked to 'sext' him at night. John felt that if she wanted to send photos, he was 'obligated' to send some, too, and would ultimately bring himself to orgasm every time she sent him pictures. This series of events typically happened 4-5 times per night, and John would be tired at school the next day. He hadn't told his mother any of this, of course. When I tried to explain to John that he was not 'obligated' to do anything, he looked at me like I had started speaking a foreign language.

When mom came back into the room, she asked how everything went. I said John looked fine, physically. She then said (out loud) that she was pretty sure he was using his phone all night, and that's why he wasn't sleeping. She asked if I had any advice for that, and I suggested something she had never thought of – take the phone away. She, too, looked at me like I had started speaking a foreign language. Poor John almost passed out as mom said that one of these days, she might just go through his phone to see what he's been doing. I never mentioned what was going on (due to privacy concerns), but I can only imagine the amount of...*material*...she found when she went through his phone. Hopefully, John learned his lesson.

Another common stereotype in medicine is anxious women. To be fair, men get a lot of anxiety, too, but the stereotype is the young woman with chest pain and trouble breathing, worried about a heart attack but actually having a panic attack. Many of the young women I have seen with these symptoms are having anxiety issues. However, I once had a young lady present with similar symptoms, but she didn't appear anxious. She said her symptoms were worse at night, which is *really* common with anxiety. When people get nervous, they sometimes hyperventilate, which leads to dizziness and shortness of breath. This woman, however, kept waking up at night *because* of her shortness of breath – she didn't wake up and *then* get short of breath. In medical terms, she had orthopnea, and that's not a common feature of anxiety. It's usually related to heart or lung issues.

While her exam was reassuring that day, I wasn't comfortable saying she had the 'stereotypical' problem. I ordered an echocardiogram (an ultrasound of the heart) and gave her some diuretics (water pills) because it sounded like she had mild heart failure. She had no swelling in her legs, and no history of heart problems, but as I said in the last chapter, trust your gut. She improved on the water pills, and the echocardiogram showed heart valve disease. Even though she was so young, she needed a valve replacement. After surgery, she was fine.

Not all stereotypes involve age or gender. In medicine, nurses and providers tend to prejudge patients based on their chief complaint. For example, toothaches and back pain are the classic red flags for 'I want narcotics.' 'Personal' issues almost always involve sexually transmitted illnesses. Other stereotypes are more subtle. People often expect that someone with a foreign-sounding name won't be fluent in English, or someone who looks or smells dirty will be uneducated. We assume all sorts of things, and while those beliefs are sometimes correct, it's important to remember that not everyone fits a stereotype. Every patient you see deserves to be treated like a person, no matter who they are. Think about where people are coming from, and remember to be courteous. Yours might be the first friendly face your patient has seen in quite a while, which is good medicine, too.

# 9

## Being Human

Believe it or not, healthcare workers are human, too. We get sick. We get depressed. We get divorced, addicted, and hurt. We get overweight. We get underweight. Sometimes we even kill ourselves. In this profession, some of those things happen more often than usual. We are always so worried about everyone else that we forget to take care of ourselves. We worry about our patients, our families, our friends and coworkers. Many of us seem to feel guilty about taking time for ourselves, but we are of no help to anyone when we are sick, hurt, depressed, or burned out. First, we need to take care of ourselves, and then we can take care of everyone else.

Since we have already talked about eating and drinking during the workday, I will be brief here. One of the main reasons people get dehydrated at work is that no one has time to refill their water jug. My solution to this problem was a giant jug – mine holds about 50 oz of fluid. I only need to fill it once per shift (okay, twice on a 12-hour day). The $10 I spent on that jug was the smartest money I've spent on my health.

There's another aspect of 'being human' worth mentioning. Human beings are social creatures by nature, despite more and more interactions becoming digital. When people come to the doctor's office, they are always scared of something, and it's okay to relate to them. While the standard in medicine is to avoid talking about ourselves, sometimes the best way to help a patient is by telling them a little bit about our own lives. Patients value our opinions, so when we say something heartfelt and relatable, it means even more.

One night, when I was in college, I had a terrible experience. Someone close to me set me up, and I was tied up with rope and shoved under a desk. There were several people involved. The whole incident took about 45 minutes, but there's a large portion of the incident I can't remember. By the end of the night, I had rope burns all over my body. I screamed so loud, for so long, that I developed a yeast infection in my throat. I had nightmares for years after that, and didn't trust anyone. In hindsight, it was pretty classic PTSD (posttraumatic stress disorder). I mention this because after recovering (thanks to Divine Intervention, a former special-ops soldier, and my wife), I could immediately recognize an abuse victim. Since then, I have cared for a handful of victims. I didn't ask them *if* they had been abused; instead, I would start our conversations with, "So, are you still having nightmares?" They were always shocked and wouldn't answer my questions until I told them my story. Once they knew I understood what they were going through, they would talk to me. I was able to help them move forward, but not until I let my walls down enough to be relatable.

Sometimes, being human means stepping out of the medical role. People who are anxious, depressed, or grieving will always benefit from a kind word. After completing the medical part of a visit (talking about meds, treatments, referrals, etc.), it's okay to put the computer down, focus on the person in front of you, and have a supportive conversation. Sometimes, just acknowledging that someone is in a difficult situation is helpful. It validates their feelings and lets them express themselves without fear of judgment. We all know how helpful that can be, and sometimes that simple validation means even more when coming from a medical professional.

Not all of this 'human stuff' is doom and gloom. I have often had the privilege of taking care of pregnant, engaged, or newlywed people. Saying 'Congratulations!' doesn't take any time and makes everyone happy. It often changes the whole tone of a visit. Sometimes, the visit changes so much after a 'Congratulations!' is spoken, it almost becomes *two* visits. For example, I saw a young woman who was pregnant, who wanted to talk about abortion options. She had only recently found out she was pregnant, and she was terrified. She was still in school, wasn't married, and everyone involved wanted her to have an abortion. She never even had the chance to decide if she was excited about her pregnancy; she was simply brought to the doctor's office.

To make matters worse, I was working in urgent care that day. This young lady was trying to have a life-changing discussion with a total stranger. After we talked about the various options for aborting a pregnancy, we talked about the support programs for new mothers. I made it clear to her that while I couldn't offer any abortive treatments that day, I was not judging and offered to help her in any way I could (referrals, talking to her parents with her, etc.), regardless of her decision.

At the end of the interview, I said, "Congratulations!" and she started sobbing. I was the only person to have congratulated her – including her family, friends, boyfriend...everyone. It was heartbreaking. By being human that day, I changed two lives. The first life changed was my patient's. We spoke to her parents before she left, changing the family dynamic for the better – at least the young lady's opinion was being considered at home now, which was a critical improvement. The second life changed was mine. Never before had someone started crying after I congratulated them. I wasn't ready for that reaction, but I learned from it. Since then, I have made a point of expressing congratulations and condolences at the start of my visits, even if they might seem out of place. The response from patients has been overwhelmingly positive. I highly recommend this approach to everyone.

There is one last point I would like to make about being human – we are not perfect. We each have our strengths and weaknesses, and we all have value. When we take care of people in a medical setting, we see them in their most vulnerable states, and sometimes we fall into the trap of feeling superior to our patients. I have an expression, "I fix mechanics, not cars." I say this because I am no better than the mechanic – he doesn't know how to fix people, but I can't fix my car. We need each other, and we should treat each other as equals. It keeps me humble. However, I also use this expression with pride. I have been teased in the past because I don't know much about cars – the stereotype being 'men love cars.' My answer is simple, "I fix mechanics, not cars." In other words, I don't need to fix my car when I can fix the mechanic, and I have no reason to feel ashamed. I love this expression because it helps keep me grounded in life. Feel free to use it!

# 10

## Moving Mountains

It's depressing how often people find themselves in unfortunate circumstances. In medicine, sometimes we are blessed with the opportunity to help move mountains for people. It usually doesn't take much work, either – a few minutes of our time can have enormous consequences for the people we are helping. For providers, the most straightforward example is referrals. Sending a patient with a severe problem to see a specialist is appropriate, but just ordering the referral and sending the patient home often results in an appointment several weeks or months later. For chronic issues, that's usually fine. Sometimes, though, people can't wait that long. In those cases, you have two options – send the patient to the emergency room or call the specialist yourself. Sending someone to the ER is easy. Too often, though, this results in a financial burden for patients, an outpatient referral, and no change in urgency for the specialist visit. To be fair, a common reason for this outcome is inappropriate ER visits in the first place. The ER is a great resource, but it shouldn't be a dumping ground.

A much more cost-effective and timely solution is to call the specialist yourself (interestingly, if you're a specialist, calling a primary care provider can have the same benefits). Most of the time, talking to a provider directly results in patients being seen within 1-2 days, or even within a few hours. For 10 minutes of your time, you can save someone thousands of dollars and weeks of pain and stress. It's like being a superhero!

On a related note, no matter what branch of medicine you go into, you will see people with anxiety and depression. These issues are so common that they are often overlooked. During a typical workday, everyone is so pressed for time that monitoring for mental health issues can fall by the wayside. Even though most offices have patients fill out a questionnaire to screen for depression, people aren't always honest, especially if they are depressed, anxious, or embarrassed. As a receptionist or a tech, alert the nurse if you see someone who looks miserable. As a nurse, be confident enough to take the initiative and assess troubled patients (or anyone else). If you're a provider, listen to what your staff is telling you, and take the extra time to ask people if they're okay. Good medicine isn't done on a schedule, no matter what anyone says. Sometimes, you have to grind your day to a screeching halt to make sure the person in front of you is okay – whether they're a patient, a coworker, or anyone else. Please, do not *ever* feel wrong for doing this. Going the extra mile for people is the hallmark of a great healthcare worker.

Even in an urgent care or ER setting, it only takes 5-10 minutes to talk to people about treatment options for anxiety or depression. I have had these conversations many times. When appropriate, I will start medications, but I always arrange for close follow-up (either with me or their primary care providers). Typically, people can't get in for primary care visits for several weeks, sometimes even months, but by going the extra mile and calling their primary care providers directly, I routinely get people onto schedules within 1-2 weeks. Doing this doesn't sound very extraordinary, but it makes a big difference for patients and their families.

Here's an unusual example of moving mountains. I once had a patient with heart failure and lung disease who had difficulty taking care of herself. She meant well, but due to some mild developmental delays, managing her medications was about as much as she could handle. Every summer, she would get overheated, have a hard time breathing, and get admitted to the hospital. She had many health problems, so it was often hard to get her breathing back under control after she decompensated. Eventually, I contacted her case manager about finding an air conditioner for this patient, so she would stop getting admitted to the hospital. I was told that insurance wouldn't cover one, and there was nothing else to be done. My response was to call the insurance company directly and work my way up the corporate chain of command until I could speak to someone with decision-making power. I then explained that they could either pay several hundred dollars for an air conditioner, or *thousands* of dollars every summer for hospital therapy. Oddly enough, she got an air conditioner and stopped getting admitted to the hospital. This task would not have been possible for the woman by herself, but it only took me an hour or two. Mountain moved.

# II

## Don't Interrupt. Seriously.

According to everything I've heard, the average time it takes for a provider to interrupt a patient after the initial "How can I help you today?" is about ten seconds. Let's take a moment and consider the implications here – someone comes to your office for help, tries to explain their dilemma, and within 10-15 seconds, they are interrupted with rapid-fire questions until they are given instructions and sent home. The odds of someone feeling happy after a visit like this are slim, especially since they are paying for it. I realize most providers are trying to stay on schedule, but we shouldn't forget that healthcare is still a service industry – and customer service matters.

Interrupting during a conversation is a common habit for people in general (ever been in a conversation?), but it happens a *lot* in health care. We tend to ask open-ended questions, then immediately redirect people to much more focused questions. Receptionists, techs, nurses, providers – everyone is guilty of this at times. Ironically, if you stay quiet, people will usually tell you everything you need to know in half the time. I have remained silent when people are angry, sad, or just plain talkative, and it works like a charm. They talk themselves out, tell you virtually everything you need to know, and save you the hassle of arguing over which details matter most. After the visit, they feel like you listened (because you did), and they go home feeling much more satisfied with their visit.

Staying silent and letting someone finish speaking is a lot harder than you think (for some people, anyway). Try it the next time you have a patient in front of you. Just stay quiet for a few seconds longer than usual. Obviously, awkward silence isn't the goal, but you want to wait long enough that the patient has to decide to either say something or not. When they finish speaking, you can steer the conversation in the direction you want it to go. This trick saves me time way more often than not, though I admit it isn't perfect. Sometimes people just don't talk. In that case, this technique won't get you far, so feel free to go back to rapid-fire questions. Just remember to let people finish their answers.

# 12

## It's Okay to Cry

Burnout has become a real problem in the medical field. While it's occasionally necessary to finish some paperwork after hours (depending on your position), I would not recommend taking your work home with you. I mean this in both a literal and figurative sense. On a literal level, don't take your patients home. Or date them. It's *really bad* for your career. On a side note, if you do end up becoming involved with one of your patients (or think you might), the responsible way to approach this situation is to transfer their care to someone else, at which point you are free to mingle.

On a figurative level, try not to let the emotional issues of your patients affect you. As harsh as it sounds, you can't save everyone. Sometimes, you can't even help everyone. The key is to do your best, be willing to move mountains when you need to, and understand your boundaries and limits. Even if you do all of this perfectly, there will still be times when you see things that are so sad or awful that you break down and cry. That's okay. Many people will tell you to 'suck it up,' or that crying is a sign of weakness. Honestly, I think they are wrong.

Near the start of my career, I was caring for someone in a hospital. It was a young woman who had been declared brain-dead, but her partner (nonmarried, different race, but truly dedicated to this woman) was unaware of her status. She was the woman who had her organs harvested the same day her partner was looking forward to seeing her again – the case from the ethics chapter. Remember that story? I mentioned that I cried right in the hospital. To clarify, I was sitting in an out-of-the-way spot, not causing any distractions or making any noise. In this chapter, I will tell you what happened next. The woman in charge of the organ donation program (we'll call her Kelly) told me I needed to 'toughen up.' However, at that point in my life, I was a black belt in two separate martial arts systems, with training in kickboxing, self-defense, sticks and knives, and grappling. I was tough already, and I still cried. When she finished speaking, I explained why she was wrong.

Crying is not a sign of weakness. It's a sign of strength. When Kelly told me to 'toughen up,' she meant that I shouldn't cry because I shouldn't feel any emotions on the job. I respect people who can distance themselves from their work, and not allow emotions to affect them. However, I'm built differently. I don't allow my emotions to interfere with my work or my judgment, but I don't avoid them, either. I embrace them. I went to work, day after day, taking care of this woman and facing the challenges involved, knowing full well that it would hurt, but I did it anyway. That's tough. That's strength and courage. I am not even remotely embarrassed by my tears – they make me human. After years of training and being overtired, overworked, and overstressed, I haven't lost my humanity. I can still empathize, and that empathy gives me the strength to keep caring for people.

When I finished explaining this to Kelly that night, she had no idea how to respond, so she walked away. The nurses who were standing nearby gave me a round of applause. When I went home at the end of my shift, I was still a little sad, but I was okay. Even now, sometimes I take care of people so unfortunate that I have to go outside and blink away tears before continuing to see patients. Years later, I still consider it a mark of strength. You should, too. Never let *anyone* belittle you for crying.

Before moving on, I would like to clarify that I don't think Kelly was a bad person. She had a hard job, and she coped with it by distancing herself to avoid being emotionally drained by her career, and there's *nothing* wrong with that. She probably thought her advice would help me. If you identify with Kelly, please understand that I respect you. The lesson in this example is to realize that crying does *not* imply weakness. However, neither does *not* crying. We all cope in our own ways. As long as we support each other, and avoid judging ourselves or each other, we can *all* do a better job for our patients. That's what a good healthcare team is all about.

# 13

## Being a Patient

People say doctors are the worst patients. Honestly, I'm pretty sure nurses are worse than we are, but either way, it's close. Everyone else in health care is pretty reasonable, but nurses and providers are terrible patients. It's hard for us to surrender control of the medical decision-making to someone else when we know the repercussions of the choices involved.

Unfortunately, I've had my share of experiences as a patient. I have had surgery (too many times), been on IV infusions, and had to wait for imaging results. The panic that patients feel when waiting for results is genuine. The fear of surgery is real. Even though I knew and understood everything going on in the operating room when they wheeled me in on a gurney, it was still overwhelming for me as a patient. Waking up from anesthesia is rough, too. I'm not willing to tell those stories because they involve absent clowns, an imaginary guillotine, and a lot of screaming. We're moving on now.

One of the most striking things about being a patient (as a healthcare worker) is the change in perception of time. While working, the usual flow of patient care seems pretty constant. You never notice if people are waiting because you're doing the best you can to keep up, regardless of the wait time. As a patient, though, you are only noticing the time people spend on *you*. The same process that feels quick as a provider (check-in, history, exam, x-rays/labs, diagnosis, etc.) takes forever as a patient. The delay between getting an x-ray and seeing the provider again can seem enormous – but we never notice because we are moving on and seeing other people during those delays. Overall, it's a humbling experience. Suddenly, you realize why people get so angry or anxious when they are in the same quiet room for an hour. It can make you feel guilty. As a patient, it gets tempting to tell your providers that you work in healthcare to get special treatment. If you choose to be that person, go for it. After all, there are perks to being in medicine, and while I generally try not to, even I have played the doctor card for myself and my family. Nobody's perfect.

As a patient, try to remember that you *don't* know best. When the health issues are your own (or those of a close friend or family member), you are too close to the situation to be objective and rational. If your provider tells you things you don't want to hear, you should still listen. If you think someone is wrong, it's okay to speak up! After all, you have medical experience, too. If necessary, get a second opinion – but if both of your providers agree, you probably need to accept what they are telling you. Be careful about researching your own conditions, too. We have all had patients that looked on the internet before coming to the office, who now believe they have ten cancers, five sexually transmitted illnesses, and that weird genetic condition no one knows how to pronounce. It's worse for healthcare workers because most of us have *seen* the horror stories we read about online. Trust me, don't ask Google for your diagnosis (though sometimes it's okay to do some research using a trustworthy source). See a real provider, instead.

# 14

## Those Endless Calls...

Have you ever chosen *not* to hire a professional because you know someone who can help you for free? When you enter the medical field, people start calling *you*. They will tell you all sorts of things, some of which you never wanted to know. The big question is how you answer. Do you have them call their doctor, or do you offer advice? It seems like an easy question to answer, right? Help your friends out, and give them advice.

However! That's not a great plan. As soon as you answer their questions, most people assume they can call you with questions at any time, and now you have a burden on your hands. There's also a lot of liability in phone medicine. If you give someone the wrong advice, they can sue you for damages. Even if the patient might not sue you, what about their family? Not to mention the idea that you might want to have a life outside of medicine. Spending your time off by giving free phone advice to your friends and family is not the healthiest hobby you can have.

Those phone calls will start early, too. I started getting questions from teachers and secretaries in college – and I hadn't even gone to medical school yet! The same thing happens to nearly everyone who goes to school for medicine – nurses, technicians, physician's assistants, nurse practitioners, therapists, etc. Sometimes, when you get bombarded by questions from people you care about, you feel guilty about not answering them, especially when you know they're anxious about something or may not have insurance. However, if you care about them, get them to someone who can help. Someone who isn't family. When the patient is someone you care about (or even yourself!), you are too close to the situation to be objective, as we discussed in the previous chapter. There is no reason to feel guilty – the best thing you can do for someone is to get them assessed by an objective provider.

I realize this can be hard to do. My personal approach, right or wrong, is to triage. I get a quick story and either advise people they can keep monitoring the issue at home, or that they need to be seen and examined. My family and friends have gotten used to it, I don't have to feel guilty, and everyone still feels like they got some advice. The liability to myself is low, and so is the risk to the patients. It's a nice middle ground.

As an aside, don't be offended if people *stop* asking you questions. Within a year or so of being married, everyone started asking my wife their health-related questions instead of me. For the record, my wife had no medical training or experience at the time. It was so blatant that sometimes people would come up to my wife and ask her questions while she was right next to me! These were friends and family! At first, I thought they were angry or intimidated, or maybe I had offended them somehow, but there was no major issue. Eventually, I realized the only change was that no one was bothering me anymore. It's been nice. Now I feel bad for my wife. Funny how life changes.

# 15

## Drug Dealing

I had a lot of good reasons to go into primary care. I had a million good reasons to get out. One of the main reasons I gave up primary care was that I felt like a drug dealer. An incredible number of people in this country use narcotics for chronic pain. There is not much evidence that it helps, either. Ironically, people tend to become *more* sensitive to pain the longer they use opiates. There are plenty of side effects, too, including constipation, nausea, and fatigue. Of course, the biggest problems with opiates are the high rates of addiction and death that we hear about in the news. Somehow, none of this stops people from wanting more opiates. Few providers like to manage chronic pain meds, so the responsibility often falls to primary care providers. As controlled substances, opiates require extra paperwork to prescribe. It takes several minutes to write a single script and document the correct information. Since a typical primary care practice consists of

3,000-5,000 patients, you will likely write a *lot* of scripts for opiates, even though 'pain management clinics' are becoming more common (at least as of the time of this writing). Trying to determine which patients need pain meds and which ones are just looking for easy drugs is a tedious process. Sometimes you will be wrong. Sometimes you will be right. Whether you give the meds or not, there is the potential for significant suffering. It's enough to keep you awake at night.

I once had a patient on opiates who was dying from brain cancer. My office received several anonymous phone calls claiming that he was selling his meds. When I asked him if he was selling his opiates, he was evasive, defensive, and angry. Unfortunately, that's a reasonable reaction from someone, whether they are innocent or not. I had to stop writing his meds. Ethically, I wasn't sure what to do. Legally, I couldn't ignore those phone calls. He confronted me in the office, asking if I would truly stop writing his pain meds when I knew he was dying. When I confirmed that I had to stop writing his meds, he stormed out, yelling that he would report me (to the state, the federal government, and all sorts of organizations that I'm not sure exist). Teaching point – when people start yelling threats, it's a great indicator that they were lying to you from the start. While he never reported me to anyone (that I know of), it was still a sad case.

Opiates aren't the only drugs people will try to sell or abuse. For example, some patients want stimulants for focus issues or attention disorders, but they can be used for weight loss, too. Sometimes people who claim to need stimulants for weight loss are secretly anorexic or bulimic. It takes a lot of time to sort through the possibilities. I once had a young man come to my office on a Friday afternoon, looking for Ritalin (a stimulant). We'll call him Paul. He was a teacher and a baseball coach who stated that his Adult ADHD was becoming a problem, as it did every spring during baseball season. Throughout the rest of the year, Paul was able to function normally. I had never seen him before, but I was suspicious because stimulants improve your reaction time, which helps if you're trying to hit a fastball. So I asked him, quite bluntly, if he was honestly going to show up asking for stimulants on a Friday afternoon at the start of baseball season, having never met me before? When Paul said, "Yes," I made him a deal. If he went for formal psychologic testing, and the psychologist felt he needed the meds, I would provide them. Surprisingly, he went for the testing and returned for a follow-up visit. However, the psychologist recommended repeating the test when Paul had stopped using recreational drugs. As a result, I refused to provide any controlled substances, and Paul never returned to my office.

There are plenty of abused medications that are not 'controlled substances.' As providers, we always have to be aware of the possibility that patients may be abusing or diverting their drugs (selling them, trading them, etc.). It's an ugly, unfortunate truth. Make sure you do your detective work, follow up with people, conduct drug testing, and stick to your guns. As an alternative, you could avoid the hassle and make it known that you don't prescribe controlled substances at all. There are several ways to approach the issue – just don't be a vending machine. Please.

Having said all that, sometimes people will surprise you. I've had several honest patients on pain meds. The one that stands out the most was an older gentleman with a *lot* of health problems. He was open about the fact that he struggled with addiction to his opiates, but said he had a lot of pain and needed the meds. A brief workup confirmed that this guy was in rough shape. In addition to his arthritic disease and other health problems, he also had a colostomy bag, meaning most of his fecal matter went through his abdominal wall into a bag that was taped to his skin. He insisted that he needed short-acting pain meds because the pills popped into his bag within four hours of swallowing them, so the long-acting meds didn't work for him. Since I didn't know him, I gave him the longer-acting meds to decrease the risk of abuse (short-acting pain meds usually give people a better 'high'). He wasn't happy, but he did everything I asked of him for about a month. When his story wasn't changing, I decided to do some investigating.

I spoke with the local specialists and found out I could do something called a GI transit time study. The short version is this – my patient swallowed some tiny metallic beads, then had x-rays taken periodically to track how fast they moved through his gut. After about four hours, the beads were in his colostomy bag. In other words, everything he had told me was true. I put him back on shorter-acting meds and documented everything carefully so that his future doctors would know he was telling the truth. He still struggled with the balance between pain control and addiction, but he was honest with me, and we had a good therapeutic relationship.

Sometimes patients force you into a corner, and you have to make hard decisions. The next example for this chapter involves a married couple on pain meds. They were quite old, and had so much arthritis that neither of them could walk normally. It was blatantly obvious they both had chronic pain. When they joined my practice, they each had their own scripts for pain meds, which I continued. The problem started soon after – I began receiving phone calls from therapists and visiting nurses, reporting that this couple would share their meds (which, since they were on the same pill, wasn't a huge medical risk). In the medical world, sharing scripts is not allowed, especially for controlled meds like opiates. After several of these complaints came in, I explained that if they didn't stop sharing their meds (or at least didn't stop telling people about it), I would have to stop prescribing them because I wasn't willing to jeopardize my license. Unfortunately, they didn't stop, and I had to stop ordering their pain meds. I felt awful about it because they weren't *abusing* the medications, but legally they forced my hand. Sometimes you will have to make hard decisions in your career, too. Be prepared.

On a final note, sometimes the people you are caring for aren't the problem. In the previous stories, the patients were the ones having issues with their controlled substances. However, sometimes the real culprits are their family members. The easy example to understand is the patient whose children are taking their pain meds. When the kids are teenagers, the solution is simple – put the meds in a locked cabinet. If the 'children' are actually adults, this problem becomes a lot harder to solve. For example, I once took care of an elderly patient on comfort care. She was involved with hospice, was dying of widespread cancer, and had a very short life expectancy. She lived at home with her adult children, who were her primary caregivers. Every week, I was told she had more and more pain, and needed more and more pain meds. Since she had dementia, I couldn't really get her side of the story. What made me suspicious was the fact that despite her kids telling me she was getting worse, her exam never changed. She had no real tenderness that I could find; no obvious cause for her pain. She didn't look like she was being abused, but something wasn't adding up. When I asked her kids if they were taking her meds, they became extremely angry and threatened to sue me. As I mentioned previously, that's a great indicator that people have been lying. I couldn't stop writing the pain meds, because my patient was truly dying and in pain. My solution was to get social workers involved, and have her transferred to an inpatient hospice unit, where she was given her meds appropriately by professional staff. The kids never sued me, my patient was taken care of, and I was no longer putting drugs into irresponsible hands. Many people would call this a win-win situation, but I still wish it had never happened.

# 16

'Tuck Them In'

Every parent knows the best time of day is that magical moment when the kids fall asleep. It doesn't matter what time it is. Typically, this moment happens soon after you tuck in the kids at bedtime. If you don't tuck them in, they come out of their bedrooms time and time again until you do. (Yes, I realize this example is grossly over-simplified, but bear with me. It's a metaphor.)

The same approach works in medicine. As a provider, this means creating a backup plan for patients during their visit. For example, someone who has had a cold for two days rarely needs antibiotics, but most people go to the doctor's office specifically to *get* antibiotics. I have seen too many cases of people having 3-4 appointments within a week to request antibiotics because they are repeatedly told by their providers, "You have a virus, no antibiotics are needed." By the time I see them, they've been sick for 7-10 days (making a secondary bacterial infection more likely), and I treat them with antibiotics, and they get better. If these patients had been 'tucked in' during their initial visit, none of the subsequent visits would have been necessary. Here's what I mean: When I see someone who has had a cold for two days and doesn't need antibiotics, I give them a timeframe. "If you're not better by Tuesday, call me, and I will send you antibiotics." By providing a backup plan, I have avoided unnecessary antibiotics without upsetting people since they won't have to make another appointment (or copay) if they don't get better within a few days. I've had very few complaints using this approach.

Sometimes 'tucking them in' involves anticipating problems. For instance, many women will develop yeast infections when they take antibiotics. Whenever I start a woman on antibiotics, I always ask about yeast infections. If she is prone to them, I send her a script to treat a potential yeast infection, which she will only use if necessary. Similarly, if someone is going on vacation and has a cold, it would be acceptable to say, "It's viral, no antibiotics today," and send them on their way. However, it's also possible to give someone a script for antibiotics and advise them not to use the medicine until a specific day (at least seven days after the onset of symptoms). It puts people in charge of their care, prevents unnecessary phone calls and visits, and makes everyone's life easier (including your own). It takes slightly longer during a visit to tuck people in, but it saves a *ton* of time overall. It's also empowering for patients, which is a good thing. The extra few minutes it takes to 'tuck in' your patients will consistently lead to happier patients and fewer phone calls. It's a win-win for everyone.

# 17

## Standing Up for Yourself

I've become increasingly convinced that our healthcare system is built on hazing. As a student, your lectures contain more information than anyone could hope to retain. After spending enough time in a classroom, you start your clinical rotations, essentially changing jobs every few weeks. This system is supposed to expose you to various fields of medicine. What it *really* does is ensure you never spend enough time at a single location to become comfortable with your duties. You end up feeling like the dumbest person in the room for the entire time you are doing rotations. After several years of this, you get a job – with yet *another* new system to learn. For doctors, it's even worse. We go to residency after school, where we do at least three more years of rotations. Every year, we get new job duties within each rotation, so we manage to feel brand new in rotations we've already done! After all of these experiences, it's understandable that many graduates have self-esteem issues, making it hard for them to stand up for themselves. Despite this, no one ever tries to change the system. The philosophy seems to be, "I went through it, so everyone else should, too." Hazing, right?

What students need to remember is that *feeling* dumb is not the same as *being* dumb. People in healthcare are (ideally) not dumb. It takes an intelligent person to keep up with our schooling and get through rotations. I've noticed, though, that when *everyone* in the class is really intelligent, some people get intimidated and lose their confidence. If this happens to you, remember that just finishing the program you are in is a huge accomplishment. Even getting *accepted* to a program in healthcare is an accomplishment – it's a competitive field at every level! Don't let self-doubt plague you because everyone else is smart – you earned your place in healthcare and you should be proud of your accomplishments!

Having confidence and standing up for yourself often go hand in hand. When you're confident, you stand up for yourself. When you stand up for yourself, you build confidence. It's a great system, but starting the ball rolling can be intimidating. People will tell you that you're wrong, even when you're not. They will blame you for things you didn't do. Even worse, the people that do these things are usually loud, aggressive, and rude. They are used to getting their way and often bully their way through life. Unfortunately, they know the new person on the job is an easy target. Don't let it happen. Never take the fall for someone else. I'm not advocating selfishness or being cutthroat. Accepting failure sets a precedent, making you a scapegoat, then a punching bag, and later a doormat.

If someone tries to blame their failures on you, make it clear that you weren't at fault. Drawing a hard line at the beginning of a new rotation/job sets you up for success by demanding respect and making it clear you won't tolerate bullying. Just remember not to be overly aggressive yourself. Forcing someone else to accept their failures will teach them to do things properly and prevents patients from being hurt by repeat failures in the future. No matter how you look at it, standing up for yourself is the right thing to do – for everyone.

One night, when I was on call at a hospital, I had a patient in the ICU. They had a severe infection, but were on the right antibiotics, and had been improving. However, when I made my rounds in the morning, I noticed that someone had recorded higher and higher temperatures for this patient all night – and no one called me. Worsening fevers in the ICU are a warning sign that something is wrong. By the time I found the problem, multiple elevated temperature readings had been recorded throughout the night. When I asked the nurses why I hadn't been notified of my patient's worsening fevers, they had no idea. They asked the staff member who had taken vital signs that night (Rachel, for simplicity) about the fevers, and she reported she had spoken to me several times during the night, and I chose not to take any actions. There you have it – I had just been blamed for someone else's failures. In this case, Rachel failed to call me, and then lied about it.

When I explained to the nurses that no one had contacted me, I showed them my phone and my pager, and nothing was there. The nurse manager then started looking into the situation, and very quickly realized that *every* patient on the unit had fevers that night, but only when Rachel was checking vital signs. Digging a little further, it was discovered that Rachel had been leaving her thermometer on the heating vent, for ease of access. Since the thermometer was warm to begin with, all of her temperature readings were falsely elevated. At that point, every single temperature reading obtained by Rachel that night had to be deleted, since the data was inaccurate. If I hadn't stood up for myself, I would have been blamed for negligence regarding my patient. Numerous patients in the ICU would likely have had their medications changed unnecessarily, which can be dangerous for people on life support. Even worse, if no one had figured out the source of the issue (leaving the thermometer on the heating vent), this would have happened again and again. In the grand scheme of life, it seems like a harmless mistake, but it had big consequences – especially because the error was covered up and blamed on someone else. Hopefully, Rachel learned her lesson before anyone got hurt.

Standing up for yourself doesn't have to be confrontational. While I prefer to deal with people directly, there are other ways to deal with bullying or harassment in the workplace. Written complaints to managers or human resource departments are a perfectly valid option for telling someone that certain behaviors are unacceptable. This method allows an aggressor to be dealt with more safely – you don't even have to be in the room at the time (unless you want to be, of course).

Another option for dealing with disagreements involves emailing someone directly, while including your supervisor/

human resource manager in the email. This strategy allows you to state your case directly, puts pressure on everyone to remain professional, and simultaneously sends a clear message to your supervisors that you are having problems with your coworker. As an added benefit, writing an email allows you to collect and organize your thoughts without having someone shout at you or interrupt you. Similarly, having a friend, coworker or manager accompany you as you talk to someone is a great way to ensure everyone remains professional and avoids bullying/harassment during the conversation. There are many ways to handle these situations, so please stand up for yourself – both in and out of the workplace.

# 18

## Take Care of Your Staff!

In medicine, similar to the military, there is a pretty standard chain of command. While in reality, insurance companies are at the top (making financial decisions that limit the rest of us), most of the time, doctors like to *think* they are in charge. They forget about things like CEOs, office managers, the board of directors, etc. However, all of that aside, they do tend to get the final say during the day-to-day provision of care. While it would be great if everyone got along nicely, with no hard feelings, no personality conflicts, no abuse of power...that's just not reality. People disagree, they sometimes resent each other, and everyone gets affected. That's why it is *so* important to take care of your staff, regardless of your 'rank' within the medical world.

The first priority of a leader is to keep things running smoothly. However, their second priority is to take care of their staff. Providers cannot function without the support of their clinical, administrative, and maintenance staff. As a provider, you have a leadership role within your team, which comes with added responsibility. You get to 'set the tone' for the workday. If you are respectful, most of your coworkers will be, too. If not, your team will probably fall apart. Remember that not everyone has to *like* each other to *work* together.

The same principle applies to everyone else. Nurses cannot function without providers, receptionists, technicians, maintenance crews, etc. Receptionists rely on nurses and providers for guidance. Every single member of the team has value. Every single member (ideally) works hard and deserves to be treated with dignity. I realize that reality isn't perfect, and sometimes problems need to be dealt with, but that can be done professionally, too. We're all on the same team, so treat everyone accordingly.

Now that the humanitarian lecture is over, let's talk about something else. If you take care of your staff, your staff will take care of you. Let me give you some examples. When I was in primary care, I had one nurse and one receptionist. It was only the three of us working in a basement. My nurse (who was supposed to retire soon) stayed with me for over a year. I bought her lunch regularly. I did my best to make things as easy for her as I could. I refused to allow her to clean up after me (sorting papers, throwing out my lunch plates, etc.). I took the same approach with my receptionist, who had minimal experience but was a hard worker and a caring person. As an aside, my nurse turned into a true blessing. When I met the woman who became my wife, she had been through a lot. It was tough to work through some of our differences at the beginning. My nurse listened to me vent my frustrations every week, which was *not* in her job description. She gave me some good advice, too. I'm sure she wasn't paid enough for that, but we were a team. I did my best to take care of her, and she took care of me.

In my career, I've gone out of my way to take care of hospital nurses, too. Whenever I admitted a patient, I would personally go to the floor and tell the receiving nurse about the patient, my concerns, and what to expect. After a few weeks of giving sign-out to the nurses, they started trying to coordinate their phone calls to me (for med orders, etc.). When I was covering the night shift, sometimes that coordination let me sleep for a few hours at a time. Again, I took care of my staff, and they took care of me.

The concept of taking care of your coworkers applies to every health center, regardless of size. While working in a large urgent care center, I had a relatively consistent team of providers, nurses, techs, and receptionists. When I could, I helped enter vital signs or print notes for the nurses. I walked to the receptionists to ask them to help me with patient issues in person, waiting in line with everyone else, instead of calling or emailing them. It made things much easier for everyone and prevented miscommunication. I routinely walked over to the x-ray techs and asked them if my orders were correct for the pictures I needed. On occasion, I walked over to the lab to ask questions, too. Even now, the added touch of asking in person, instead of via email or phone, makes a big difference. It helps everyone on the team feel appreciated, which is good for morale. It also keeps me from getting bored since I'm always doing something. That's important, too.

# 19

## Documentation. It Matters. A Lot.

I teach my students and trainees (as medical providers) to write their notes with several goals in mind. The primary objective is to document what happened during a visit, so you and your partners can continue to care for people without having to start over at every appointment. When writing notes, remember that patients can read them if they choose (so no condescending language in the notes!). The most crucial reason for detailed notes, though, is for the jury. Should you ever be sued in your career, your only defense will be your notes. While I haven't been sued yet (as of this writing), I have been threatened with hundreds of lawsuits. Yes – *hundreds*. Remember, people can sue you for anything, even if you've done nothing wrong.

Years ago, I saw a patient who had recently been diagnosed

with a viral illness by another provider in our group. She had seen several different providers in a short amount of time. While that may have been convenient for her, it made finding a diagnosis difficult because no one could see how her symptoms evolved – each provider saw only a single snapshot of her illness. As it turned out, she developed pneumonia but didn't receive treatment until it was severe. She did fine overall but made a formal complaint to the insurance company. Based on my documentation, the insurance company determined that my actions were appropriate and removed me from the complaint. I'm not sure what happened to the other providers, but being removed from those proceedings is a *huge* relief.

My next example involves someone I saw with a clear-cut case of appendicitis, which is an emergency and requires surgery. I had no difficulty making the diagnosis and recommending the proper treatment (going to the hospital for surgery). The problem, in this case, was the patient, who refused to go to the emergency room. He didn't believe me when I said he needed emergency surgery. I tried for almost 20 minutes to convince this person to go to the hospital, even told him he could die from this, but he wouldn't go. I documented the conversation in detail (it was a long note), and he went home. Several months later, I was informed that this person had gone to the hospital two days after I saw him because his pain had worsened. He was taken straight to the operating room for surgery because he had a ruptured appendix. He was trying to sue me, claiming I had misdiagnosed him with 'constipation.' However, when his attorney looked at my note from that day, the case was dropped because I had practically begged this man to go to the hospital. Once again, my notes saved me from serious harm before I even knew there was an issue.

As you can probably tell by now, I write longer notes than a lot of my colleagues. It used to slow me down, but it's much less of a problem in today's world. I use a microphone and medical software to dictate my notes. I still have to proofread them before I sign anything (you would not *believe* the mistakes the software can make), but it still saves me a ton of time, and my notes are better than they used to be. Good documentation is essential for nurses, receptionists, and technicians, too. Every single patient interaction, including a phone call, needs to be documented carefully. While these notes are often shorter, they are just as crucial. If you have trouble typing quickly (since more and more practices are now using electronic medical records), try dictating instead. The technology is readily available. No matter how you approach documentation, please make sure you are thorough. It will save your career more times than you realize.

## 20

Check Your Ego at
the Door

One of the scariest things in the medical world is pride. It can be as deadly as germs, antibiotic resistance, cancer, even politics. In moderation, pride can be a good thing. People who take pride in their work will try their best to do a good job. However, a healthcare worker who is too proud to ask for help might hurt or misinform their patients. Someone who makes an error may be too embarrassed to apologize, preferring to cover up their mistake, which can be disastrous for patients in the long run. By checking your ego at the door, you mentally accept the idea that you don't know everything, so it's okay to look things up, ask for help, etc. That kind of humility will help you be a great healthcare worker. The following examples are not glamorous, funny, or earth-shattering, but they all help illustrate how important it is to be humble.

Knowing your limits is probably the most important skill you can have in healthcare. The most dangerous person on the team is the one who *thinks* they know what they're doing, but won't ask for help. Ideally, no one should ever get upset about being asked for assistance. I realize our world is not ideal, but I would much rather risk being yelled at for double-checking with someone than risk hurting a patient. Always ask for help if you need it, or even if you think you *might* need it. This principle applies to everyone on the healthcare team. Receptionists should feel free to ask any nurse or provider about patients they are checking in. Nurses should feel comfortable asking providers to help triage an unusual case. Providers should feel like they can ask for help without being judged. I approach people at every level of our health center with questions. If *I* can ask questions as a physician without losing credibility, *everyone* should feel comfortable asking for help.

When I transitioned from primary care to urgent care, I befriended a physician assistant with decades of experience in the emergency room. We came from very different backgrounds, but urgent care is a balance of primary care and emergency medicine. Even though I (technically) outranked him in the medical world, his knowledge and experience in emergency medicine were invaluable to me. Instead of pretending I didn't need any help, I asked him questions every day until I was comfortable with the more emergent issues we encountered. Since we help manage many more chronic issues in urgent care than in the emergency room, he started asking me questions, too. Together, we became the anchor-team for our urgent care center, and we both improved our skills significantly. None of that would have been possible if we were too proud to ask each other for help.

Many healthcare workers, especially providers, find it difficult to admit they don't know something. In contrast, I am perfectly comfortable telling people I don't know the answers to their questions, but I will do my best to find the information they need. In those cases, I will do a quick literature search to find the answer, if possible, or call a specialist for advice. Sometimes, I explain that *nobody* knows the answers they're looking for because medical science just isn't there yet. On the rare occasion that I have no idea how to help someone, I admit it plainly, "I'm sorry...I have no idea what your diagnosis is, but I will get you to the right person for help." I then (personally) contact the right specialist to have my patient seen as soon as possible. I have never had a single person complain while using this approach. People might not be happy when their doctor doesn't have the answer, but everyone appreciates honesty.

The last topic I want to address regarding humility in healthcare involves apologies. When someone is at the doctor's office, they are scared of something, so when a patient has a bad outcome (whether we made a mistake in their care or not), they can flip from nervous to angry quite quickly. This happens to both patients and providers, but we as healthcare workers need to be the ones to step back and be calm. I have witnessed multiple situations play out predictably. A patient gets upset (for whatever reason). The staff then gets defensive, which makes the patient even angrier, and then an argument starts. Ultimately, both parties go home angry and upset. When something like this starts to happen, an apology can quickly deescalate the situation and make all the difference.

As soon as I make a mistake, I admit it, correct it, and apologize. Sometimes I send a script to the wrong pharmacy (or forget to send it at all). Sometimes, I forget to order an x-ray, and a patient is stuck waiting in a room for an extra 20-30 minutes before I realize the issue. In those circumstances, I put the order in, tell the x-ray tech (in person) that I forgot to order the x-ray, and ask them to take care of my patient next. I then talk to the patient, admit that I forgot to order the x-ray, and explain that I spoke to the techs, and they will be next in line. I always say that I am sorry, too. People are understandably annoyed, but they have never complained about me (to my knowledge) because I 'owned' the mistake, corrected it, and apologized.

Sometimes I am asked to step in when someone else has made a mistake. For example, patients are occasionally mis-labeled as 'checked out' and the computer system no longer shows that they are waiting for a provider. What ends up happening is the patient gets forgotten in the exam room because no one knows they are still in the building. When they come out of their room to complain about their wait time, everyone scrambles, and the patient gets mad. My response is to tell the patient that I will see them next. When I go into the room, I explain what happened and apologize on behalf of the staff. It doesn't fix the problem, and I never reveal who made a mistake, but I take responsibility and apologize. If no one made a mistake, there's nothing wrong with saying, "I'm sorry that happened to you." Apologies are such simple things, and they cost nothing to give, but pride is too often in the way. Please, check your ego at the door. You can accomplish so much more without it.

# 21

⧉

# Faith Matters: God Cures, We Help.

This is a controversial topic in today's world, but that doesn't make it less important. I am a Christian. I realize not everyone is, and that's okay. There's no judgment here, but since I am the one writing this book, I am going to give you my perspective. Every day, I have the opportunity to do God's work. I help people, and it feels wonderful. As you have seen in this book, healthcare is not always sunshine and rainbows, but the good days *far* outnumber the bad. I always try to remember, though, that I am just helping. Before we had modern medicine, most people did okay. Not *great* (which is why the life expectancy was so much shorter in ancient times), but okay. To stay humble, I remind myself that God heals, and I just help. When I have patients who disclose to me that they are Christian, I tell them this. The rest of the time, I keep it to myself.

I am not recommending that you share your religious beliefs with your patients (though you are certainly allowed to if you choose), but don't forget them. They serve as a moral compass, helping you remember why you went into healthcare. If you are not religious, just remember the values you brought with you to medicine. My faith is my greatest source of strength, compassion, perseverance, and success. Whatever you believe in, I hope it brings you the same.

# Final Thoughts

Thank you for making it all the way to the end of this book! I hope you learned something on this little journey. I would like to reiterate that everything here is a compilation of my own thoughts, opinions, theories, experiences, and education. Not everyone will agree with everything I have written, and that's okay. If all I accomplish is to get people thinking about these issues, I will have accomplished a lot. My goal is to help people learn the *art* of healthcare, and as we all know, art is very subjective. Still, I hope these little lessons prove helpful to you in the future. If nothing else, I hope it was entertaining!

# Credits

After years of learning and personal experience, I have no hope of giving credit everywhere it's due, but I will try. If you played a role in my education, please accept my sincere thanks. To my family members and friends who supported me along the way, I thank you, too. If you happen to be the nurse who stayed with me for over a year, please know that you will have a special place in my heart forever. You are a big part of the reason I got married. I would like to thank my wife for helping me find myself again. Most of all, I thank the Lord for being with me every day, helping me on my journey through life. Finally, I want to thank everyone who reads this book and gets even a *single* gem of wisdom from it. Please carry these lessons with you into the future. No, seriously - I'm going to be old someday, and I'm going to need help. Someone will have to take care of my wife and I, so please remember these life lessons!

\*\*\*\*

God bless you all.
I wish you all the best.
- Dr. Mike -

www.ingramcontent.com/pod-product-compliance
Lightning Source LLC
Chambersburg PA
CBHW030300030426
42336CB00009B/460

* 9 7 8 1 7 3 6 8 3 2 9 1 2 *